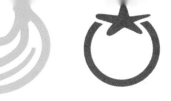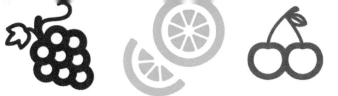

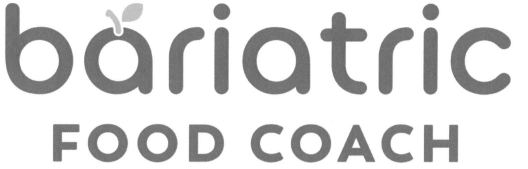

bariatric
FOOD COACH

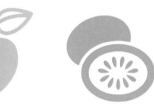

Focus
Challenge
WORKBOOK

Steph Wagner MS, RDN

Welcome

Welcome to the Bariatric Food Coach Focus Challenge! I am so excited to have you join me and all the many others who are ready to refocus with you. The challenge runs three times a year for a four-week period. This workbook is meant to supplement the online material that you can find on the Focus Challenge Page when you are logged into BariatricFoodCoach.com. You can also use your smart phone camera to scan QR codes inside this workbook to find additional videos or material on the website. You can practice now with the QR code below that will take you to the Focus Challenge Page!

I will communicate challenge information over email (double check your spam folder or email support@bariatricfoodcoach.com if you are not receiving emails from me). I will also keep the challenge page updated.

There are four live calls on Zoom that I hope you can attend. The replay is always available the next day, if you cannot join live. Our first live call is a Goal Setting Workshop before the challenge begins. The other three calls are coaching calls where I focus on the theme of our challenge and you can connect with other members taking the challenge.

In the following pages you will find more information about what the challenge is, an area to fill in important dates and information, a place to take notes during our Goal Setting call and the Goal Tracker where you will write in your goal and follow along.

Along the way I hope to encourage you to be kind to yourself, stay positive, have fun and do not worry about being perfect. Setting clear goals can really build confidence and help you feel more like yourself again!

Cheering you on,

Steph
steph@bariatricfoodcoach.com

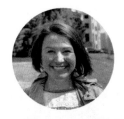

Table of Contents

BARIATRIC FOOD COACH FOCUS CHALLENGE WORKBOOK

What Is the Challenge?

One of the most common questions members ask me when it comes to the challenge is "what is it exactly?"

On this page I want to give you insight into why I created these challenges, what they are, and what they are not. We hear the term "challenge" quite often in our diet culture. If you hear the word challenge and think of weight loss challenges, sit up challenges or even boot camps, try to wipe those more intensive ideas away. This is a 'focus' challenge, which is more about finding a specific goal to lean into, instead of losing X amount of pounds by X date.

What the Focus Challenge is:

A four week period to focus your mind on one healthy habit.

Each person's goal is unique to them. One person may need to focus on water. They find that staying hydrated helps them with late-night snacking. How to stay hydrated day in and day out for a month is the challenge for that person. Other healthy choices 'overflow' (pun intended) from their goal.

The challenge is a time to ask yourself what you need most.

One person may realize they need to focus on sleep habits the most.

One person may realize they need to focus on meal planning the most.

One person may realize they want to really challenge themselves to keep a detailed food diary.

All of these are great goals, however, the real challenge is to pick ONE of those goals. It may be tempting to pick water, meal planning and food journaling but that would not be a focused goal. More on that later.

What Is the Challenge?

What the challenge is not:

A weight loss challenge.

The goals are not about the scale.

Sure, you want to experience weight loss if you are trying to lose, regain, or continue your weight loss after surgery! However, we are focusing on the actions and not just the results. Focusing on your one goal will overflow to other areas of your life. You'll notice healthier choices coming easier with a focused goal and the scale, OR your clothes, OR your energy, OR your pictures will show results. I will talk more about the scale later in the workbook but for now remember what the challenge IS and what it is not.

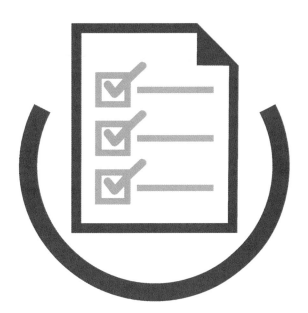

Important Dates

Important Dates and Info (fill in the blanks)

Go to  to see the list of dates.

This Challenge runs _____ to _____

The theme of this Challenge is: _____
_____

What the theme means to me: _____
_____

The live Goal Setting Workshop is:
_____

The live coaching calls with Steph are:
1- _____ , 2- _____ , 3- _____

Goal Setting Workshop Notes

Clear Goals - goals have these three things :

i. _____

ii. _____

iii. _____

Week One Excitement

i. Set your goals with _____ in mind

ii. Keep it simple and specific

iii. Some will want to 'reset' for week one

    1. Keep the overall goal of the challenge to _____

iv. If you have been way off track and are wanting to do a big push on getting carbs out in the first week, be prepared to _____

_____.

v. Avoid pushing yourself really hard on _____ during the first week if you are feeling 'fuzzy' from getting carbs down!

DISCLAIMER

"A diet 'reset' is not necessary. Getting back to basics is a great way to start the challenge. If you like the idea of doing a little 'reset' type of diet to clear your mind, remember it is not changing the size of your pouch. Nothing special is happening except getting your body used to lower carbohydrate amounts and refocusing your mind. Avoid weighing yourself as it can lead to yo-yo dieting." - Steph W.

Notes from Live Goal Setting Call

It's All about the Goal Tracker

(see page 10)

Goal need to have 3 things :

i. Do a brain dump of all the possible habits you'd like to focus on

_____

_____

_____

_____

ii. Go back and circle the ones that feel most important

iii. Below, brainstorm how you can turn that into a goal

_____

_____

_____

_____

iii. Some things to consider as you choose your goal

1. Sit on your goal before you commit! Why? _____

2. Cornerstone Goals are _____

3. You should feel some _____ about your goal

4. _____ and _____ goals are more likely to be finished

It's All about the Goal Tracker

(continued...)

iv.   Sample Goals :

1. Journal my foods before the day starts, 4 days a week
2. Drink 80 ounces of water, 5 days a week
3. Avoid eating after dinner, 5 nights a week
4. Plan meals every Sunday night, allow 1 night for takeout
5. Avoid popcorn or chips for 4 weeks
6. 20 minutes of walking, 4 days a week

 If it doesn't challenge you,
it won't change you.

\- Fred Devito

Goal Tracker

Below is the image for the Goal Tracker for the whole challenge. You can choose to check the boxes and take notes on this page, or you can use the weekly view of the tracker for each week later in the workbook. Or you can do both!

28-DAY CHALLENGE GOAL TRACKER

FOOD GOAL (F)

EXERCISE GOAL (E)

PRIZE

bariatric
FOOD COACH

DAYS TO ADD-ON:

WEEK ONE

	MON.	TUE.	WED.	THURS.	FRI.	SAT.	SUN.
F	☐	☐	☐	☐	☐	☐	☐
E	☐	☐	☐	☐	☐	☐	☐

WEEK TWO

	MON.	TUE.	WED.	THURS.	FRI.	SAT.	SUN.
F	☐	☐	☐	☐	☐	☐	☐
E	☐	☐	☐	☐	☐	☐	☐

WEEK THREE

	MON.	TUE.	WED.	THURS.	FRI.	SAT.	SUN.
F	☐	☐	☐	☐	☐	☐	☐
E	☐	☐	☐	☐	☐	☐	☐

WEEK FOUR

	MON.	TUE.	WED.	THURS.	FRI.	SAT.	SUN.
F	☐	☐	☐	☐	☐	☐	☐
E	☐	☐	☐	☐	☐	☐	☐

I go over the goal tracker in more detail during the goal setting workshop. You'll pencil in your food-related goal, your exercise-related goal and your prize (that you will treat yourself with at the end of the challenge!) You will follow along with the boxes next to food and exercise to check if you hit your goal.

Simplify and Declutter

You've simplified your goals. Yay!

Now take a moment to think about your simplified goal and how you can declutter things in your life to help your goal feel simplified. Let's take meal planning for example.

If your goal is to meal plan, do you have a simple strategy on how to make that happen? If you have cookbook and notebook and saved recipes in one spot and magazines somewhere else, now is a good time to declutter your meal planning system. Do you like to write your meals out on a written calendar but have your recipes all saved on a Pinterest board? Great!

Then clear out the rest. Determine your strategy and declutter anything that distracts that strategy. This will help you stay focused and keep it simple. If water is your goal but you have a cupboard full of water bottles, spend time clearing out that cluttered area and determine which one or two water bottles you will truly use. If you have a pantry full of flavored water packets, clear those out too and determine if you really like them or not. Restock the ones you know will help you drink more water and get rid of the others!

When we declutter physical things, our brains feel less cluttered. Your goal will start to feel more tangible, more doable and simplified.

How can you declutter to help you simplify and stay focused on your goal?

_____

_____

_____

_____

_____

Positive Thinking

It may sound cliché, but never underestimate the power of positive thinking! There is a famous book with that very title if you'd like to read more. If you decide this is a goal you can do and visualize how you will do it and what it will feel like when you do, you are focusing on positive thinking. "Stinking thinking" is easy to slip into. The negative thoughts will try to come in that you're too busy, it's too hard, your family isn't supportive enough, you always give up and so on. When those thoughts creep in, identify them as stinking thinking and validate what you are feeling. "Of course this is hard! Of course I am tired. Yes, I am really busy. But I can do hard things and I can simplify this to make it work and will feel better if I do."

What positive affirmations can you use to encourage yourself in your focus challenge?

_____

_____

_____

_____

Use the QR below for a link to positive quotes and scriptures

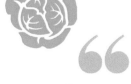

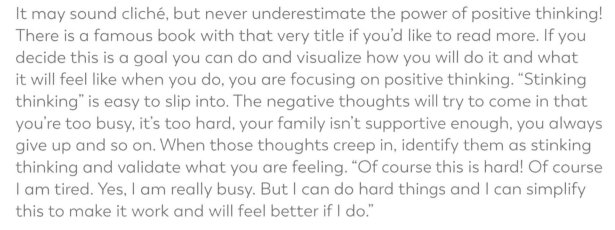

" It does not matter how slowly you go as long as you do not stop.

- Confucious "

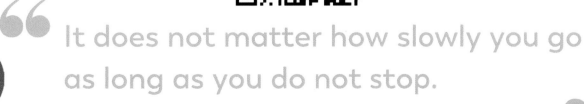

Meal Planning

Everyone has their different styles of meal planning and some seasons of life your planning style may need to change. Maybe your goal is specific to meal planning but even if it is not, there is a good chance your goal still needs some amount of planning to make it happen. If your goal is to not snack after dinner, you'll want to have a good plan for dinners so that you are full and satisfied from your meal and able to find something else to do in the evenings.

The website is full of meal planning resources! If you like following a fully written meal plan, you'll enjoy the meal plans page on the site. If you instead tend to eat the same breakfast and lunch but need just dinners planned, try one of the 'dinners' menus on the site. If instead you like to have a list of quick meal ideas for the Season, I have a guide for that. If you like browsing all the recipes on the website and saving them for later, use the Collections feature on the site. If you want ideas on what popular grocery stores have to offer, check out the Grocery Store Guides. Use your Smart Phone to take a photo of the QR code below for the meal plans list and click/tap Meal Planning on the top menu for a list of additional resources.

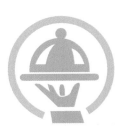

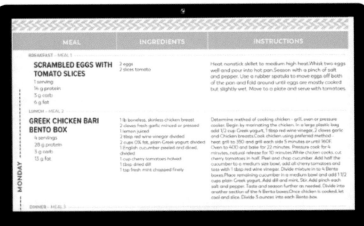

Water

Water is an awesome cornerstone goal and many of you will decide to make it your main focus. Yay! When you are more hydrated, your hunger is better controlled and energy more even through the day. Many have found making water their goal improves their food choices. That is why it is such a powerful goal!

How much water?

The recommendation for water is to drink one ounce for every kilogram of body weight. For those us who use pounds, that means we **divide our current weight by 2.2**. If that is an overwhelming amount of water to you, aim for 96 ounces a day. If you are nowhere near that, try for a minimum of 64 ounces a day.

What counts as water?

Every program differs but I say follow the three C's. If it's not caffeinated, not carbonated and under 15 calories (per 8 ounces) you can count it as water. This includes herbal tea, flavored water packets or squirts, fruit infused waters, broth, homemade popsicles and so on. I personally love a warm seasonal herbal tea in the evenings. *Note: Programs differ on artificial sweeteners. I personally try to use natural no-calorie sweeteners (example: Stevia) when possible.

What are some of your favorite ways to get in water?

_____

_____

_____

_____

_____

Exercise

When you start adding in exercise, it can bring up a lot of questions about eating. If you wonder if your eating plan should or shouldn't change with your exercise routine, check out the members video course on the website entitled "Exercise and the Bariatric Diet" or use the QR code below.

Something to keep in mind is when you work out at a less intense, lower heart rate (like a walking pace that allows you to carry a conversation) you burn more from fat and less from carbohydrates. This tends to help control hunger as well. While higher intensity workouts are great for cardiovascular (heart) health, it can drive up your hunger. If you start running or other higher intensity cardio workouts, keep an eye on if you find yourself hungrier for starchy foods.

As you think about your exercise goal for these next four weeks, visualize how it's going to work. What will you do? Where will you do it? When is it most likely to happen? Answer those questions in the space below.

Our Community

One of the best parts about being a member and doing a challenge is the community that comes with it! It is such a gift to connect with others from all over working towards healthy habits and on similar paths (though different journeys) from yours.

There are three main ways to connect with the Bariatric Food Coach Community

Small Groups

Small Groups
in GroupMe

Inside the GroupMe app are several groups based on surgery time, timeline and/or special interests. If you haven't joined a group already, you can find a link on the challenge page or in the top navigation click on Members Resources then Get Connected then Smaller Groups.

Facebook Group

Closed Group
in Facebook

The Facebook Group is also a great way to connect with even more members. There you will find threads about what goals people are setting and what they are doing to make it happen. It's an encouraging and inspiring place to be!

Live Calls

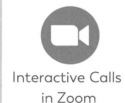

Interactive Calls
in Zoom

We will have three live calls on Zoom during the challenge where you can connect with others live in the chat box, ask me questions live and hear some coaching on the challenge's theme. If you cannot make it live, the replay will be available the next day.

Links to join the live call will be emailed and posted on the Facebook group page. Refer to the dates for the live calls you wrote in on page 5.

Finishers and Prizes

If you are wondering if you submit your goal anywhere or if you report to me, the answer is yes...and no!

At the end of each week, I will email out a link to a form. If you completed the goal you set out to do, you will fill out the form. Each person's first name and first initial of their last name will go on that week's "Finishers Board." I also draw prizes from the finishers to keep things fun and exciting!

 Every accomplishment starts with the decision to try.

\- John F. Kennedy

Because of the number of participants in the challenge, you will not submit to me a report of each day or your goal tracker. Instead, you can use the small groups on GroupMe or the Facebook group to share your goals, a snapshot of your tracker and/or your progress. You are also welcome to email me a request to look at your food journal if you would like some ideas or feedback.

I also recommend keeping follow-ups with your bariatric dietitian for more individualized nutrition care. If you need help finding a dietitian, email me and I will find someone licensed in your state and specializing in bariatric surgery.

Week One

WEEK ONE

FOOD GOAL (F)

EXERCISE GOAL (E)

WEEK ONE

	MON.	TUE.	WED.	THURS.	FRI.	SAT.	SUN.
F	☐	☐	☐	☐	☐	☐	☐
E	☐	☐	☐	☐	☐	☐	☐

Takeaways from Week One:

_____

_____

_____

_____

_____

Notes from Live Coaching Call #1

The theme for this challenge is:

_____

_____

_____

_____

_____

_____

_____

_____

_____

_____

_____

_____

_____

_____

The Scale

We tend to be hard wired to have expectations around the scale and what we think it should do. If you have four days of getting back to basics and following a really healthy eating plan and the scale says you lost three pounds already, you are pumped! If you repeat those same four days and you gain a half a pound, you are annoyed and confused.

This is because the scale is not the best method of measuring progress. We just think it is.

Sure, we walk into the doctors office and the first thing they do is have you step on a scale! Your body weight does have clinical significance in a medical chart (it's how they can give you the appropriate dose of medicine for example) but beyond your medical chart, does it really tell you much? While we do want to see the scale go down after surgery, we also know it will go up, down, left and right on any given day and the bigger picture is more helpful than daily or even weekly weighing.

My recommendation? Keep the scale under your bed or on the top shelf of a closet and pull it down for a once a week weigh in. Try not to fixate on the number too much, notice it and release it and think of all the many, many other ways to measure progress.

Look at photos, notice your clothing, realize your endurance is increasing, cross your legs and smile at the changes. Watch your labs improve, tie your shoes more comfortably, enjoy compliments from those who know you well and all the many other non-scale victories that remind you that healthy habits do amazing things. The progress is much more multi-faceted than a number on the scale.

What are the ways you like to measure success outside of the scale?

_____

_____

_____

Week Two

WEEK TWO

FOOD GOAL (F)

EXERCISE GOAL (E)

WEEK TWO

	MON.	TUE.	WED.	THURS.	FRI.	SAT.	SUN.
F	☐	☐	☐	☐	☐	☐	☐
E	☐	☐	☐	☐	☐	☐	☐

Takeaways from Week Two

_____

_____

_____

_____

_____

Notes from Live Coaching Call #2

The theme for this challenge is:

_____

_____

_____

_____

_____

_____

_____

_____

_____

_____

_____

_____

_____

_____

Be Okay with the Gray

A popular theme for one of our past challenges was 'be okay with the gray.' This means even the best set plans will have to change. Maybe you wrote out a meal plan that was so cut and dry but when life started it didn't look so cut and dry after all. Maybe you had a 30 minute walk planned but instead you had to walk a parking lot in between a doctor's appointment and a grocery pickup! Perhaps you said you wouldn't snack after dinner but you found you needed a deli meat and cheese stick rollup in the evening after all. This is all being okay with the gray! Life is not black and white. Instead of being hard on yourself when things look differently than you'd planned, see the positive of how you adjusted, stayed flexible and stayed in tune to yourself.

What are some examples of times you embraced being okay with the gray?

_____

_____

_____

_____

_____

_____

_____

_____

Revisit the Goal

Now is a great time to re-visit the goal!

If you haven't heard me say it already, you have full permission to change, modify or adapt your goal. Do not feel married to a goal that isn't quite right after all. It is better to make a change that builds up your confidence than hold a goal over your head (that you gave yourself) and feel badly when you aren't doing it anymore.

If food journaling was your goal and it turns out you're just not into it, change your goal to water. If your goal is water but you aren't making it all the way to 96 ounces, change your goal to 80 ounces. Don't give up...modify!

What is your current goal?

_____

_____

Do you need to make any changes? If so, what?

_____

_____

_____

_____

 Aim for success, not perfection.

- David D. Burns

Week Three

WEEK THREE

FOOD GOAL (F)

EXERCISE GOAL (E)

WEEK THREE

	MON.	TUE.	WED.	THURS.	FRI.	SAT.	SUN.
F	☐	☐	☐	☐	☐	☐	☐
E	☐	☐	☐	☐	☐	☐	☐

Takeaways from Week Three

_____

_____

_____

_____

_____

Notes from Live Coaching Call #3

The theme for this challenge is: _____

_____

_____

_____

_____

_____

_____

_____

_____

_____

_____

_____

_____

_____

_____

_____

_____

Positive Accountability

     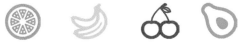

Accountability can be a really helpful and powerful tool when making behavior changes! However, it can be really delicate because we are human and there are days when we are not going to hit the goal. Sometimes we look to someone else to 'hold us accountable' but that person can easily be felt as food police if they take it too far!

This is why I call it positive accountability. If I plan to go for a walk but I don't tell anyone and I don't write it down, I don't have accountability. If I tell my spouse that I'm going to walk and he needs to make sure that I do, then I don't walk and he gets on to me, I am not going to feel positive and he won't either!

Instead, positive accountability to walk might be walking with a friend. If you have it scheduled with someone, you feel accountable to not cancel. If finding a friend to walk with is not easy (schedules, distance) see if you can find a friend to text a picture to when you are out on your walk, and she texts you hers. It's positive because you are doing it together! Should the day come that you can't walk, she may not be too hard on you but also ask when you can reschedule.

I call these kinds of friends 'people of peace.' These are the people who feel safe to ask for help being accountable to do the things you said you can do. It could be sending them a text before you walk into a restaurant and that you'll send them a picture of what you order. This also lessens the intensity of the person you are having dinner with looking over your shoulder! Positive accountability often comes from a safe, small community with one person or a couple others. Our GroupMe smaller groups are a great place for positive accountability.

Also note, you can email me at steph@bariatricfoodcoach.com if you'd like me to look over your food journal. Some members like accountability of knowing someone is going to be looking and I am happy to do that for you!

Who are some "people of peace" you could seek for some positive accountability?

_____

_____

Limiting Beliefs

A limiting belief if something you are believing that may actually be holding you back.

We all have them. The trick is identifying them and then challenging the thinking.

This was a theme for a past challenge and at the time my limiting belief was that it was just too hard to consistently exercise when you're a Mom to young children.

Some of that was true, it IS really hard to exercise when you're in a time demanding season (and not sleeping the best) but I also noticed other Moms I knew had found ways to consistently exercise. What was I believing about exercise that told me I couldn't do it during this Season of life? I started asking Mom friends what they do. When do they do it? How do they make it work? How often? One Mom took both her kids in a double stroller for a long walk. Another Mom went when her husband got home form work. I was able to push past my limiting belief and see that consistent exercise as a Mom could happen but I needed to redefine what consistent exercise meant.

Others had limiting beliefs that questioned if they could really stay on track more than two weeks or that they weren't strong enough to not snack at night. One members shared her limiting belief was that she would never find peace with food.

Once we named the limiting belief, we were able to get to work challenging the thinking!

What limiting beliefs are you believing that might be holding you back?

_____

_____

_____

_____

Week Four

WEEK FOUR

FOOD GOAL (F)

EXERCISE GOAL (E)

WEEK FOUR

	MON.	TUE.	WED.	THURS.	FRI.	SAT.	SUN.
F	☐	☐	☐	☐	☐	☐	☐
E	☐	☐	☐	☐	☐	☐	☐

Notes

_____

_____

_____

_____

_____

Support
in your home

Support at home is a really complicated topic. I am a firm believer that you should feel supported on your home turf. The truth is, it can be really complicated.

Perhaps you have a family who was supportive in the beginning but somewhere along the way, they stopped being so supportive and they didn't realize it. Or maybe your family member was never on board.

Maybe your family is fine with you eating differently but they don't want to change anything themselves leaving your home environment covered with temptation.

I wish there was a simple answer here. What I have found helpful in these conversations is to ask others how they do it. Get as many ideas and suggestions as you can. This is **phase one** and it gets your wheels turning.

In phase two, you allow yourself some space to really think through your situation. Some suggestions you were given in phase one won't work for you. Other suggestions may work in some ways but need to be tweaked. In phase two, I like to go for a long walk (or a long drive) and think through the problem. What is bothering me? What are some possible solutions?

Maybe you need to organize the pantry to put your items at eye level and all the tempting items in dark colored containers with a lid. You aren't telling your family no, but you are working towards setting up a better home turf for yourself.

Maybe your spouse really loves fudge stripe cookies but you struggle with them in the house. On your long walk you may decide you can buy fudge stripe cookies once a month for him but let him know when they're gone they won't be restocked until next month. This might help you to not get into his stash knowing that he would notice! You aren't telling him no, you're just trying to problem solve some things for your health.

Support

What problems are you facing on your home turf in regards to your health goals? Who can you ask for ideas? How can you get some space to think?

_____

_____

_____

_____

_____

_____

_____

_____

_____

COME TOGETHER

Support
in the bariatric community

Great news. Finding support in the bariatric community is better than ever! As a bariatric dietitian for over a decade, I have seen firsthand how much support has grown in this field. Support groups can be found at most all programs and many offer online options now. As a member you have access to our monthly live calls! There are Instagram pages, Facebook groups, online symposiums, and more.

The trick is to find the ones that fit you best and cut out the rest. Too much of anything can be too much! If you find you have followed too many Facebook groups, it may be worth the time to unfollow and declutter to only stay in the ones that feel most supportive.

It is also really helpful to know yourself well and what your personality needs most with community. You may like the smaller groups we have in the GroupMe app because you text with a smaller group of people. That may not be your thing and you'd prefer to follow tips on Instagram. Know that support in the bariatric community is ready and available to you, whatever your style and wherever you are. You are certainly always welcome in our Bariatric Food Coach Community!

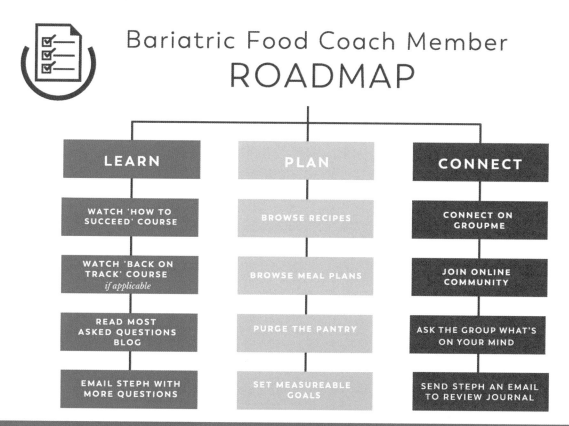

Bariatric Food Coach Member
ROADMAP

LEARN	PLAN	CONNECT
WATCH 'HOW TO SUCCEED' COURSE	BROWSE RECIPES	CONNECT ON GROUPME
WATCH 'BACK ON TRACK' COURSE *if applicable*	BROWSE MEAL PLANS	JOIN ONLINE COMMUNITY
READ MOST ASKED QUESTIONS BLOG	PURGE THE PANTRY	ASK THE GROUP WHAT'S ON YOUR MIND
EMAIL STEPH WITH MORE QUESTIONS	SET MEASUREABLE GOALS	SEND STEPH AN EMAIL TO REVIEW JOURNAL

Finishing the Challenge!

The finish line is the most exciting part! Often times we feel more excitement in the first week but as we get towards the end of the challenge those early feelings have faded. Then you realize the finish line is nearing and you are going to make it!

If you are on track to hit your goal, start planning now for your prize! Did you write down a prize on your goal tracker? Start your shopping! Add it to your cart, browse your options, get excited for the prize you will get for yourself!

If you are not on track to hit your goal, I have great news.

There is a 'days to add on' section on the goal tracker! Try not to overcomplicate this box, it is good news. This box is like someone who needed an extra semester or two in college to finish their degree. Just because they took a 'victory lap' doesn't mean they didn't earn their diploma!

Here at the Bariatric Food Coach Focus Challenge, you are allowed to finish your goals in a victory lap! If you were four walks short of your goal, put the number four in the days to add on box and each time you take a walk (even if the challenge is over) tally it up until you hit four. You can still post to your group that you finish the goal and cash in your prize. If you snacked a few nights more than you planned, it's okay! Add on a couple of days and don't sell yourself short for hitting your goal a week later. Remember, we are okay with the gray!

Notes

_____

_____

_____

_____

_____

_____

_____

_____

_____

_____

_____

_____

_____

Notes

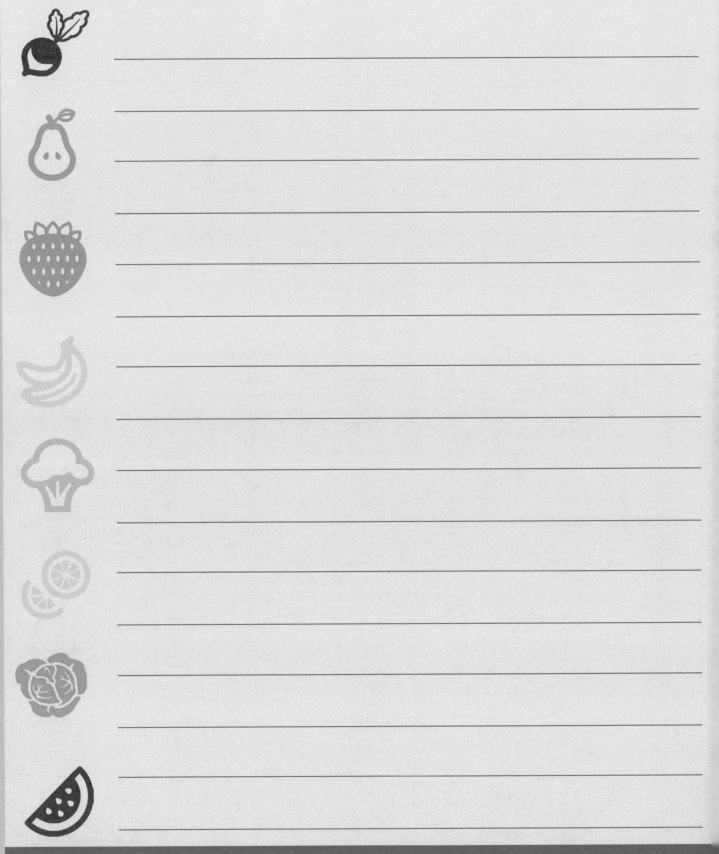

Thank you for joining me in the Bariatric Food Coach Focus Challenge! I hope it has been life-giving to you as you build habits to support your health and wellbeing. Remember to encourage yourself first and then think through any roadblock you might be facing. Be your own biggest cheerleader instead of your own worst critic!

The challenge may be over but the resources, education and support are always available to you on Bariatric Food Coach. You can email me anytime at steph@ bariatricfoodcoach.com

One additional resource I would like to mention if you have enjoyed this journal format is a 30 day workbook by my friend and colleague, Cassandra Golden Sampson. Her book "30 Mindful & Instinctive Thoughts to Start Your Day" is available on Amazon and asks great questions to help you think through your food life.

All my best to you and yours!

Steph

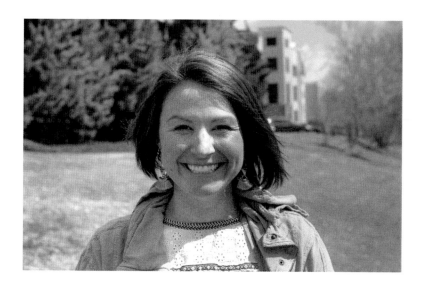

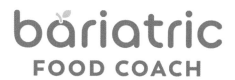

Made in the USA
Middletown, DE
05 February 2023

24127856R00022